The information provided in this book is designed to provide
helpful information on the subjects discussed. This book is not
meant to be used, nor should it be used, to diagnose or treat any
medical condition. For diagnosis or treatment of any medical
problem, consult your own physician. The publisher and author
are not responsible for any specific health or allergy needs that
may require medical supervision and are not liable for any
damages or negative consequences from any treatment, action,
application or preparation, to any person reading or following
the information in this book.